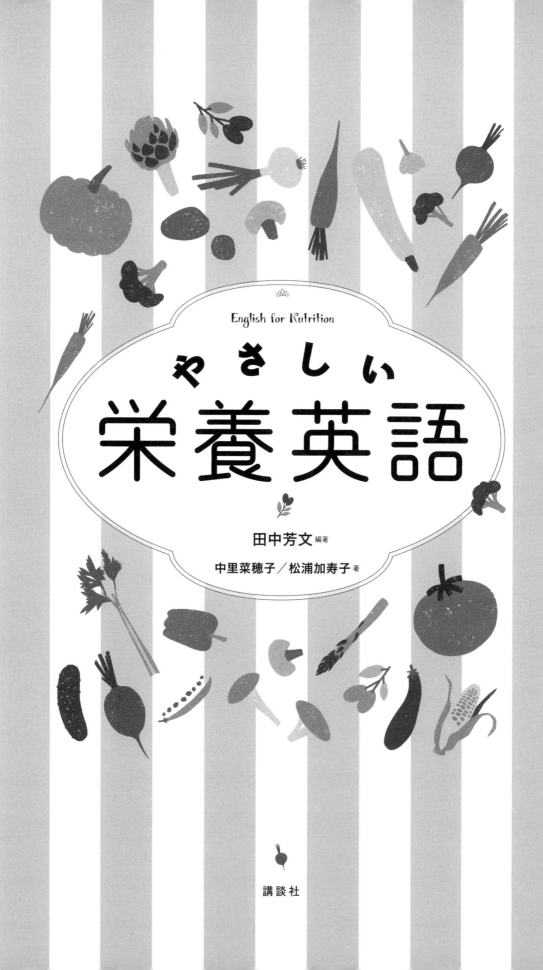

装幀：相京厚史 (next door design)　本文イラスト：北原志乃

執筆者一覧

※田 中 芳 文————島根県立大学　人間文化学部　教授　（1, 2, 5, 10, 11, 12, 13, 14, 15）
中里菜穂子————聖徳大学　語学教育センター　非常勤講師　（3, 4, 6）
松浦加寿子————倉敷市立短期大学保育学科　准教授　（7, 8, 9）

五十音順，※は編著者。（　）内の数字は担当Unit。

あらかじめご了承ください

・本書は全国の大学・専門学校で教材として使用されているため，練習問題の解答や日本語訳は付属していません。

・本書の紹介ページに，音声データが用意されています（収録箇所：各Unitの🔊の部分）。

紹介ページのアドレス
https://www.kspub.co.jp/book/detail/5134146.html

はじめに

　本書は，はじめて専門分野の英語に接する栄養学専攻の学生，および現代人の食生活や栄養に関心のある一般の人たちを対象にした英語テキストです。初心者にさまざまな専門分野をわかりやすく紹介するFor Dummiesシリーズの2冊，Carol Ann Rinzler著 *Nutrition for Dummies* (6th edition) とMichael J. Rovito著 *Clinical Nutrition for Dummies* から抜粋した，食事，カロリー摂取，食生活，栄養素，消化，摂食障害，食物アレルギー，食物汚染などに関する英文を素材にしています。

　Unit 1〜4, 6〜9, 11〜14は，まず予習としてVocabulary Checkに取り組んでください。英文にはできる限り多くの注を付けて，なるべく辞書を引かなくても読み進めることができるようにしてあります。練習問題は，A（書き取り）とB（英文整序）から構成されています。また，Unit 5, 10, 15は，少し構成を変えて，語彙，適語補充，英文和訳の練習問題に加えて，それ以前の4つのUnitに出てきた重要表現・構文・語彙の復習ができるように工夫しました。

　本書を利用することによって，食生活や栄養に関するみなさんの知識が深まると同時に，英語の学力が向上することを願っています。

　最後に，本書出版の意義にご理解をいただいた講談社サイエンティフィクに敬意を表しますとともに，出版のためにご尽力くださった同社の小笠原弘高さんにこころより感謝申し上げます。

2018年晩秋
編著者

本書は第3刷時に各ExerciseやReviewのBの一部を更新しています。

目次 contents

Unit 1 **The ABCMVs of Eating**
食事の基本 —————————————————————————— 1

Unit 2 **Determining Whether Your Diet is Adequate**
あなたの食事は適切か ————————————————————— 4

Unit 3 **Keeping Caloric Intake in Check**
カロリー摂取を管理する ———————————————————— 7

Unit 4 **Spicing up Your Life with Variety**
食生活に一味添えよう ————————————————————— 10

Unit 5 **What's a Body Made of?**
+Review　からだは何でできている？ ———————————————— 14

Unit 6 **Knowing Your Nutrients**
栄養素を知ろう ———————————————————————— 17

Unit 7 **Energizing Nutrients: Proteins, Carbs, and Fats**
エネルギーの源：タンパク質，炭水化物，脂肪 ————————— 20

Unit 8 **Aiding in Body Function: Vitamins and Minerals**
身体機能を助ける：ビタミンとミネラル ———————————— 23

Unit 9 **Water: The Most Important Nutrient**
水：最も重要な栄養素 ————————————————————— 27

Unit 10 **Binge Drinking: A Behavioral No-No**
+Review　むちゃ飲み：絶対にやってはならない行為 ———————— 30

Unit 11 **Digestion: One Step at a Time**
消化：一歩ずつ着実に ————————————————————— 33

Unit 12 **Eating Disorders**
摂食障害 ——————————————————————————— 37

Unit 13 **Food Allergies**
食物アレルギー ———————————————————————— 42

Unit 14 **Controlling Food Contamination**
食物汚染を食い止めよう ———————————————————— 47

Unit 15 **The Father of All Vitamins: Casimir Funk**
+Review　ビタミンの父：カシミール・フンク ——————————— 51

Unit 1 The ABCMVs of Eating
食事の基本

Vocabulary Check

（　　）に入る語を下から選びなさい。

1. (　　　　　) meat　赤身の肉
2. (　　　　　) grains　全粒穀物
3. (　　　　　) fat　飽和脂肪
4. (　　　　　) vitamin　合成ビタミン
5. (　　　　　) oil　硬化油
6. (　　　　　)　栄養素
7. (　　　　　)　乳製品
8. (　　　　　) food　加工食品
9. (　　　　　) meals　調理済み食品
10. alcohol (　　　　　)　アルコール過剰摂取

> abuse, dairy, hydrogenated, lean, nutrient, prepared, processed, saturated, synthetic, whole

Track01

Here's a fact that many people have a hard time believing: Eating more like your ancestors did (fresh, seasonal varieties of fruits and vegetables, lean meats, whole grains, and yes, even saturated fats) is actually better for your health and well-being than dining on some power smoothie chock-full of synthetic vitamins. (Apparently Mom and Grandma really did know best!)

Most of the time, the simplest food is also the healthiest. For example, are hard-boiled eggs a better source of fat and protein for you than a synthetic protein powder blend with some form of hydrogenated oil? You betcha.

Introducing a common-sense diet

The answer to living longer and healthier is actually as simple as A, B, C, with a couple of other letters thrown in:

- ☐ **Adequacy:** Are you getting sufficient vitamins and minerals from your food? The key here is to eat foods that are packed with nutrients rather than foods that offer nothing other than empty calories. An easy way to do this is to eat colorful fruits and vegetables, whole grains, and lean meats.

- ☐ **Balance:** Are you getting enough food from each food group? For most of your meals, you want to have more vegetables and fruits on your plate than any other type of food, such as bread, meat, or dairy.

- ☐ **Calorie control:** Are you consuming the right amount of calories — not too many or too few — per day? A great way to control calories is to limit the amount of high-sugar and high-fat foods you eat, like soft drinks, candy, cookies, and other baked goods.

- ☐ **Moderation:** Are you sure that you're not getting too much of one thing over another? When it comes to moderation, you also want to limit the amount of highly processed food you eat, like fried snack foods, fast food, and prepackaged prepared meals.

- ☐ **Variety:** Are you eating a varied diet and not the same thing over and over again? Try eating something different for breakfast, lunch, and dinner every day. Don't be hesitant to eat something you never tried before. Remember: Variety is the spice of life!

If you can answer "yes" to the preceding questions, your diet is probably one that gives you the nourishment necessary to help prevent illness and early death. That's it. Nothing spectacular. No pills. No bells. No whistles. Just plain, old-fashioned common sense.

Be wary of any product or regimen that guarantees you can live a longer, healthier life by taking a pill or supplement alone. The key to living longer and living healthier is a healthy diet and a lifestyle that incorporates regular exercise and refrains from tobacco use, alcohol abuse, or any other risky behavior.

Notes

have a hard time 〜ing／なかなか〜できない　ancestor／祖先　well-being／幸福　dine on 〜／食事に〜を食べる　power smoothie／パワーフルーツスムージー　chock-full of 〜／〜でぎっしり詰まった　apparently／どうやら〜らしい　most of the time／ほとんどの場合　protein／タンパク質　synthetic protein powder blend／合成タンパク質粉末ブレンド　You betcha.／そのとおり（＝ You bet (you).)。　common-sense／常識的な　as simple as A, B, C／非常に簡単な　a couple of 〜／2つの〜　throw in 〜／〜を付け加える　adequacy／十分さ　sufficient／十分な　be packed with 〜／〜でいっぱいの　rather than 〜／〜よりむしろ　nothing other than 〜／ただ〜だけ　empty calorie／エンプティカロリー（タンパク質，ビタミン，ミネラルなどの栄養素をほとんど含んでいないカロリー）　food group／食品群　than any other 〜／他のどの〜よりも　A such as B／たとえばBのようなA　consume／消費する　per day／1日につき　high-sugar／糖分の高い　high-fat／高脂肪の　baked goods／焼き菓子　moderation／適度　when it comes to 〜／〜のこととなると　prepacked／パック詰めされた　over and over again／何度も何度も　be hesitant to 〜／〜することを躊躇して　preceding／前述の　nourishment／栄養物　That's it.／そこが重要だ。　spectacular／豪華な，目を見張る　No Pills. No bells. No Whistles.／（薬やサプリメントなどの）錠剤は必要ない。余計な飾りもいらない（bells and whistles には「必須ではない付加物，安っぽい装飾品」の意味がある）。　plain／明白な，わかりやすい　old-fashioned／古風な　common sense／常識，良識　be wary of 〜／〜に警戒している　regimen／養生法　guarantee／保証する　live a long, healthy life／長く，健康的な人生を送る　incorporate／組み入れる　refrain from 〜／〜を控える，我慢する

Exercise

A 音声を聴いて，次の英文の（　　）内に適語を記入しなさい。また，完成した英文を日本語に直しなさい。

Track02

1. The children were hungry (　　) (　　) (　　) (　　).

2. I like cooking with olive oil (　　) (　　) butter.

3. There were large electrical goods (　　) (　　) television sets and washing machines.

4. I said it to myself (　　) (　　) (　　) (　　).

B 和文に合うように，（　　）内の語句を並べかえて英文を作りなさい。

1. ジョンはその状況になかなか対処することができなかった。
   (with, time, had, the situation, a, dealing, hard, John).

2. 料理のこととなると，メアリーは専門家だ。
   (cooking, an expert, to, when, is, comes, Mary, it).

3. 誰もが健康的で豊かな生活を送ることを望んでいる。
   (life, productive, a, to, healthy, live, everyone, and, wants).

Unit 2 Determining Whether Your Diet is Adequate
あなたの食事は適切か

―――― Vocabulary Check ――――

（　　）に入る語を下から選びなさい。

1. essential (　　　　　　) 必須栄養素
2. (　　　　) 食物繊維
3. body (　　　　) 体組成
4. (　　　　) 炭水化物
5. (　　　　) 脂肪
6. (　　　　) タンパク質
7. health (　　　　) 健康転帰
8. (　　　　) 毒性
9. (　　　　) 不足，欠乏
10. (　　　　) guideline 食生活指針
11. professional (　　　　) 専門家の勧告

> carbohydrate, composition, deficiency, dietary, fat, fiber, nutrient, outcome, protein, recommendation, toxicity

🔊 Track03

In the context of diets and nutrition, *adequacy* essentially means that your food choices provide all the essential nutrients, calories, and other mainstays of a healthy diet, including fiber and water. In other words, are you getting what you need from your diet to maintain a healthy lifestyle?

What's important to note about adequacy is that not everyone has the same nutritional demands. What is adequate for one person is not necessarily adequate for another. Usually gender, age, activity level, and body composition determine individual adequacy levels. For general guidelines for the average adult, see Table.

Table	Nutritional Needs for the Average Adult
Nutrient	*Percentage of Daily Diet*
Protein	15—20%
Fat	25—30%
Carbohydrates	50—60%
Water	Men: 3 liters (13 cups) per day
	Women: 2.2 liters (9 cups) per day

To determine whether your diet is adequate, simply track what you eat over the course of a week; then break down your meals into the main nutrient categories (carbohydrates, fats, proteins, vitamins, minerals; see the later unit "Knowing Your Nutrients" for details). Also keep track of how much water you drink.

If you see that you are consistently getting too much or too little of one of those categories, your diet may be inadequate.

Balancing your diet

Usually, the more variety in the foods you eat, the more balanced your diet will be. By eating a balanced diet, you ensure that you get the appropriate amounts of nutrients in the right proportion. Doing so allows for optimum health outcomes and helps you avoid any type of toxicity (too much) or deficiency (too little) of one type of nutrient or another.

The term *balance* also relates to variety, in the sense that you should balance your diet according to a nutritional guideline. Varying guidelines exist, and each gives you a sense of what you should be eating and in what amount in order to achieve balance.

In the context of ABCMV (refer to the earlier unit "The ABCMVs of Eating"), eating a balanced diet ensures that the types of foods you eat are in balance, and it safeguards you from having too much of one nutrient over others. Many dietary guidelines and professional recommendations go beyond this and state that you shouldn't eat too much (overconsume) fat, sugar, and/or alcohol. They suggest you eat these foods in moderation.

Notes

adequate／十分な，適切な　nutrition／栄養(摂取)　adequacy／十分，適切さ　mainstay／頼みの綱，大黒柱　in other words／言い換えれば　not everyone ～／（部分否定で）すべての人が～とは限らない　one／（anotherと対応して）一方の　not necessarily ～／必ずしも～ではない　track／追跡する，たどる　over the course of ～／～の間に　break down A into B／AをBに分類する　for details／詳細については　keep track of ～／～の経過を追う　consistently／終始一貫して，変わらず　inadequate／不適切な，不十分な　the more ～, the more balanced ～／（the＋比較級, the＋比較級で）より多くの～ほど，ますますバランスの取れた～　ensure／確実にする　appropriate／適切な　allow for ～／～を可能にする　optimum／最適の，最高の　term／用語　relate to ～／～と関連がある　in the sense that ～／～という意味で　according to ～／～に従って　nutritional／栄養上の　in order to ～／～するために　refer to ～／～を参照する　in balance／バランスの取れた状態で　safeguard A from ～ing／Aが～することから守る　one／（othersと対応して）一つの　go beyond ～／～をしのぐ，～より優れている　overconsume／過度に飲み食いする　and/or／およびまたは（両方とも，またはいずれか一方）　in moderation／適度に

Exercise

A 音声を聴いて，次の英文の（　　）内に適語を記入しなさい。また，完成した英文を日本語に直しなさい。

🔊 Track04

1. (　　　　)(　　　　)(　　　　), he was fired.

2. Water can be (　　　　)(　　　　)(　　　　) hydrogen and oxygen.

3. It is difficult to (　　　　)(　　　　)(　　　　) what she is doing.

4. Everything was done (　　　　)(　　　　) the rules.

B 和文に合うように，（　　）内の語句を並べかえて英文を作りなさい。

1. それは必ずしも悪いことではないかもしれない。
   (thing, necessarily, be, that, bad, may, a, not).

2. ジョンは酒を飲めば飲むほど暴力的になった。
   (violent, he, John, more, the, drank, more, became, the).

3. メアリーは子どもたちが寝る前に会おうと早く帰宅した。
   (before, to, they went to bed, order, the children, came home early, in, Mary, see).

Unit 3 Keeping Caloric Intake in Check
カロリー摂取を管理する

Vocabulary Check

（　　　）に入る語を下から選びなさい。

1. caloric (　　　　　) カロリー摂取
2. weight (　　　　　) 体重増加
3. weight (　　　　　) 体重減少
4. (　　　　　) 消費
5. (　　　　　) activity 身体活動
6. (　　　　　) 高脂肪の
7. (　　　　　) ナトリウム
8. (　　　　　) （病的な）肥満
9. high (　　　　　) pressure 高血圧
10. health (　　　　　) 健康問題

> blood, consumption, gain, high-fat, intake, issue, loss, obesity, physical, sodium

🔊 Track05

　Your recommended caloric intake is dependent upon your sex, age, and level of activity or exercise. For example, a healthy male in his 20s who exercises ten hours a week requires a higher caloric intake than an elderly female who is bedridden.

　Depending on what your health goals are (weight gain, weight loss, or maintaining your current weight), you need to adjust your energy consumption and expenditure to achieve that goal. Monitoring how much you're eating, what you're eating, and how much physical activity you get in a given day is important to maintain optimum health. Use this equation to estimate how many calories you should be consuming in a given day and to determine whether you need to adjust how much you're eating:

Energy In (calories consumed) − Energy Out (calories expended) =
Change in energy stores (excess/loss/equilibrium)

If you end up with a value above 0, you are eating more energy than you are burning, which means that you are building up energy in your body and thus gaining weight. If the value is below 0, you are burning more energy than you are consuming, and you are losing weight. If the value is at 0, you are neither building up energy nor losing it. You reached an energy equilibrium, which is how you maintain your current weight.

The Energy In (calories consumed) and Energy Out (calories expended) values are dependent on very important demographic variables such as age, exercise level, gender, and daily physical demands. Remember, not everyone needs the same amount of calories per day.

Many people struggle with maintaining a healthy weight, and one of the main reasons is excess calories (the Energy In component of the equation). Here are a few things to watch out for to avoid eating too many calories:

- ☐ Snacking while watching television
- ☐ Eating too many high-fat foods
- ☐ Consuming too much sugar in soft drinks

Following the "everything in moderation" rule

To avoid excesses or shortages not only in caloric intake but also in nutritional levels, the rule is to do everything in moderation. When you do things in moderation, you avoid excess or extremes. Dietary moderation refers most commonly to moderating the consumption of sinful culinary pleasures like sugar, salt/sodium, fat, and alcohol. The focus on these items in particular is due to the fact that chronic overindulgence in any of them can result in adverse health outcomes, including obesity, high blood pressure, and other health issues.

Notes

keep 〜 in check／〜を管理する，〜を抑制する recommend／推奨する be dependent upon〜／〜による，〜次第である require／必要とする bedridden／寝たきりの depend on 〜／〜による，〜次第である maintain／保つ current／現在の adjust／調節する expenditure／消費 achieve／達成する monitor／管理する，観察する in a given day／ある(特定の)日に optimum／最適な equation／方程式 estimate／推定する consume／消費する determine／決める whether 〜／〜かどうか calories consumed／摂取されたカロリー calories expended／消費されたエネルギー store／貯蔵，蓄積 excess／過剰分 equilibrium／均衡 end up with 〜／結局〜になる value／値 build up 〜／〜を蓄積する thus／ゆえに，だから neither A nor B／AでもBでもない demographic variable／人口統計学的変数 A such as B／たとえばBのようなA not everyone 〜／（部分否定で）すべての人が〜とは限らない per day／1日につき struggle with 〜／〜に苦労する excess／余分な watch out for 〜／〜に注意する avoid／避ける snack／軽食をとる "everything in moderation"／「何事もほどほどに」 shortage／不足 not only A but also B／AだけでなくBも nutritional／栄養の the rule is 〜／守られるべきことは〜 extreme／極度，極端 dietary／食事の refer to 〜／〜を指す moderate／適度にする sinful／罪深い culinary pleasures／おいしい食べ物 in particular／特に due to 〜／〜のため，〜が原因で the fact that 〜／〜という事実 chronic overindulgence in 〜／〜に慢性的に溺れること result in 〜／〜という結果になる adverse／逆の health outcome／健康転帰（病気の予防や治療の結果生じる健康状態） including 〜／〜を含む

Exercise

A 音声を聴いて，次の英文の（　　）内に適語を記入しなさい。また，完成した英文を日本語に直しなさい。

🔊 Track06

1. How much I exercise (　　) (　　) (　　) my schedule.

2. We (　　) (　　) (　　) over thirty thousand dollars in sales.

3. I know (　　) French (　　) German.

4. The word "it" (　　) (　　) "his dog."

B 和文に合うように，（　　）内の語句を並べかえて英文を作りなさい。

1. その栄養士は，その食事プランがクライアントの栄養ニーズを満たしているかどうかを判断するだろう。
   (the meal plan, will, meets, whether, the client's dietary needs, determine, the nutritionist).

2. 果物は，ビタミンだけでなく食物繊維も提供する。
   (vitamins, provide, also, only, fiber, not, but, fruits).

3. 彼が不健康なのは，タバコを吸いすぎるという事実が原因だ。
   (too much, smokes, that, due, the fact, is, he, to, his bad health).

Unit 4 Spicing up Your Life with Variety
食生活に一味添えよう

=== Vocabulary Check ===

(　　) に入る語を下から選びなさい。

1. (　　　　　) 収穫
2. (　　　　　) 小麦
3. (　　　　　) 大豆
4. (　　　　　) 薬味, 調味料 (塩・胡椒, ソースなど)
5. (　　　　　) food　異国風の食べ物
6. (　　　　　) amount　適切な量
7. food (　　　　　) 食物源
8. dietary (　　　　　) 食事療法
9. (　　　　　) store　食料雑貨店, スーパーマーケット
10. (　　　　　) salad　付け合わせのサラダ

> appropriate,　condiments,　exotic,　grocery,　harvest,　regimen,　side,
> source,　soy,　wheat

🔊 Track07

　　The world we live in provides a bountiful harvest of foods to eat. Yet, even though literally tens of thousands of foods are available, people usually confine themselves to eating no more than maybe a hundred or so, and the diets of the vast majority of people are created from about 20 or fewer of all the items available.

　　If you sit down and tally what you eat, you'd probably be surprised at the simplicity of your own diet. Think about it. What do you normally eat?

　　Chicken, beef, and/or pork? Wheat, rice, soy, and/or corn? A few other fruits and vegetables? Perhaps some fish?

　　People's diets tend to be very plain and boring. Chances are you know at least one person, maybe a few (maybe even you), who goes to a restaurant and orders the same thing or makes the same meals time and time again at home. Perhaps Tuesday night is pot roast night, and Friday night is pizza or take-out Chinese night.

But opting to put different condiments on a pot roast isn't really diversifying your diet. To change things up, add something truly different. Try a new protein source, opt for fruits and vegetables you don't generally eat, experiment with new-to-you herbs and spices. In addition to your pot-roast-and-potato mainstay, for example, go for the tilapia with creamed kale or roasted duck with mango salsa once in a while. *That's* diversity.

People often opt for a non-diverse diet because of convenience and familiarity. Whipping up something familiar for dinner is less time-consuming, and choosing the same things when you eat out eliminates the possibility of being disappointed in your selection. Yet your diet's diversity depends on the availability of exotic foods and your willingness (and ability) to add them to your dinner plate. By varying the foods you eat, you ensure that you're getting the appropriate amount of nutrients from your food source.

A quick and easy way to broaden your dietary regimen is to try something different — a new food you've never had before or a menu selection you don't generally make — for each meal for a week. For example, eat some star fruit (found in most grocery stores) with oatmeal in the morning instead of strawberries. Or for lunch, opt for the grilled vegetable panini with a side salad instead of the usual burger and fries. For dinner, go ahead and eat a vegetable you may have distanced yourself from when you were a child. You still may not like it after all these years, but you may get lucky and discover your next favorite food!

Notes

spice up ～／～に（香辛料で）一味添える，～をよりおもしろくする　provide／与える，供給する　bountiful／たくさんの　yet／しかし　even though ～／～ではあるが　literally／文字通り　tens of thousands of ～／何万もの～　available／手に入る　confine oneself to ～／～に限定する　no more than ～／たった～，ほんの～　maybe／もしかすると　～ or so／～かそのくらい　vast majority of people／大半の人々　tally／計算する，数え上げる　probably／ことによると，もしかしたら　be surprised at ～／～に驚いている　simplicity／シンプルさ　Think about it.／ちょっと考えてみてください。　normally／普通は，通常は　and/or／およびまたは（両方とも，またはいずれか一方）　perhaps／たぶん，十中八九は　tend to ～／～する傾向がある，～しがちである　plain／味気ない　boring／うんざりするような　chances are ～／たぶん～であろう　at least／少なくとも　time and time again／何度も何度も　pot roast／ポットロースト（蒸し焼きにしたローストビーフ）　opt to ～／～することを選択する　diversify／多様に変える　protein／タンパク質　opt for ～／～を選ぶ　generally／普通は，通常は　experiment with ～／～を試す　new-to-you／よく知らない，使ったことのない　in addition to ～／～に加えて　pot-roast-and-potato mainstay／ポットローストとポテトが主食の食事　go for ～／～を選ぶ　tilapia／ティラピア（アフリカや中東でよく食される鯛に似た白身魚）　creamed kale／ケール（濃い緑の葉物野菜）のクリーム煮　roasted duck／鴨のロースト　mango salsa／マンゴのサルサ（刻んだトマト，タマネギ，チリから作られた，メキシコ料理につけるソース）　once in a while／時々，たまに　That's diversity.／それこそが多様性だ。　non-diverse／多様性のない　because of ～／～のために，～が原因で　convenience／便利さ　familiarity／親しみのあること　whip up／手早く作る　time-consuming／時間のかかる　eat out／外食する　eliminate／取り除く　possibility／可能性　be disappointed in ～／～にがっかりする　selection／選択　depend on ～／～による，～次第である　availability／入手の可能性　willingness／意欲　ability／能力　add A to B／AをBに加える　by varying the foods you eat／色々な種類のものを食べることで　ensure／確かなものにする　nutrient／栄養素　broaden／広げる　star fruit／スターフルーツ，ゴレンシ　oatmeal／オートミール（押し麦のおかゆ）　instead of ～／～のかわりに，～ではなくて　grilled／網焼きの，グリルした　panini／パニーニ（具材をパンではさんだホットサンドのようなイタリアの食べ物）　burger and fries／ハンバーガーとポテトフライ　go ahead and ～／お先に～してください　distance A from B／BからAを遠ざける　after all these years／何年たっても　get lucky／ついている

Exercise

A 音声を聴いて，次の英文の（　）内に適語を記入しなさい。また，完成した英文を日本語に直しなさい。

🔊 Track08

1. I am not losing weight (　　　　) (　　　　　　) I stopped eating sweets.

2. Japanese students (　　　　) (　　　　　　) be shy in English conversation class.

3. (　　　　) (　　　　) (　　　　　) three meals a day, I eat a lot of snacks during the day.

4. My mother was so (　　　　　) (　　　　　　) my grades.

B 和文に合うように，(   )内の語句を並べかえて英文を作りなさい。

1. 塩と胡椒をスープに加えてください。
   (the soup, to, please, salt and pepper, add).

2. キャンディの代わりに新鮮な果物を選びましょう。
   (fruit, candy, choose, of, fresh, instead).

3. どうぞ先に召し上がってください。
   (and, go, please, eating, ahead, start).

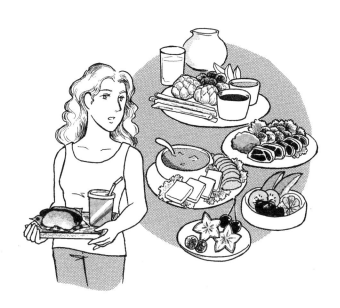

Unit 5: What's a Body Made of?
からだは何でできている?
+Review

🔊 Track09

Sugar and spice and everything nice... well, more precisely water and fat and protein and carbohydrates and vitamins and minerals.

On average, when you step on the scale, approximately 60 percent of your weight is water, 20 percent is body fat (slightly less for a man), and 20 percent is a combination of mostly protein, plus carbohydrates, minerals, vitamins, and other naturally occurring biochemicals.

Based on these percentages, you can reasonably expect that an average 140-pound person's body weight consists (1) about

- ☐ 84 pounds of water
- ☐ 28 pounds of body fat
- ☐ 28 pounds of a combination of protein (up to 25 pounds), minerals (up to 7 pounds), carbohydrates (up to 1.4 pounds), and vitamins (a trace)

Yep, you're right: Those last figures do total more than 28 pounds. That's because "up to" (as in "up to 25 pounds of protein") means that the amounts may vary from person to person. Ditto for minerals and carbohydrates.

Why? And how? Because <u>a young person's body has proportionately more muscle and less fat than an older person's, and a woman's body has proportionately less muscle and more fat than a man's.</u> (2) a result, more of a man's weight comes from protein and muscle and bone mass, while more of a woman's weight comes from fat. Protein-packed muscles and mineral-packed bones are denser tissue than fat.

Weigh a man and a woman of roughly the same height and size, and his greater bone and muscle mass means he's likely (3) tip the scale higher every time.

Notes

be made of ～／～でできている　sugar and spice and everything nice／砂糖やスパイスや素敵なものすべて（英語の童謡(nursery rhyme)の一節 "What are little girls made of? Sugar and spice And everything nice"から）　precisely／正確に　on average／平均して　scale／体重計　approximately／おおよそ　body fat／体脂肪　slightly／わずかに　naturally occurring／自然発生する　biochemical／生化学物質　based on ～／～に基づいて　reasonably／合理的に　140-pound／約63.5キログラムの　84 pounds／約38.1キログラム　28 pounds／約12.7キログラム　up to ～／（数値が）～まで　25 pounds／約11.3キログラム　7 pounds／約3.2キログラム　1.4 pounds／約0.6キログラム　trace／ほんの少し　yep／（口語で）yes　figure／数字　total／合計～となる　vary／変化する　ditto for ～／～も同じ　proportionately／比例して　bone mass／骨量　-packed／（複合語で）～のぎっしり詰まった　dense／密な　roughly／およそ　muscle mass／筋肉量　tip the scale／重さがある

Exercise

A 英文中の次の語を日本語に直しなさい。

1. fat (　　　　　)
2. protein (　　　　　)
3. carbohydrate (　　　　　)
4. muscle (　　　　　)
5. tissue (　　　　　)

B 英文中の (　) 内に入る語を下から選びなさい。

1. (　　　　)
2. (　　　　)
3. (　　　　)

> to,　of,　as

C 下線部を日本語に直しなさい。

Review (Unit 1〜Unit 4)

A 英文の（　）内に入る語を下から選んで記入し，英文を日本語に直しなさい。

1. The cooler was packed (　　　) bottles of water. (Unit 1)

2. See the bottom of this page (　　　) details. (Unit 2)

3. Is there anything (　　　) particular you want to do tomorrow? (Unit 3)

4. It will cost (　　　) least 700 dollars. (Unit 4)

> in, for, at, with

B 和文に合うように，（　）内の語句を並べかえて英文をつくりなさい。

1. 彼女はその新しい仕事を引き受けることを躊躇していた。(Unit 1)
   (accept, was, the, she, job, hesitant, new, to).

2. 適度にアルコールを飲むことは君の健康にとってよいかもしれない。(Unit 2)
   (your health, moderation, good, alcohol, in, be, drinking, for, can).

3. 健康は食べるものに左右される。(Unit 3)
   (you, on, your health, the food, depends, eat).

4. 朝食を用意するのに10分しかかからなかった。(Unit 4)
   (breakfast, than, to, 10 minutes, it, prepare, more, took, no).

C 次の英語を日本語に直しなさい。

1. synthetic vitamin　　（　　　　）ビタミン
2. essential nutrient　　必須（　　　　）
3. processed food　　（　　　　）食品
4. body composition　　体（　　　　）
5. vitamin deficiency　　ビタミン（　　　　）
6. calorie intake　　カロリー（　　　　）
7. sodium　　（　　　　）
8. obesity　　（　　　　）
9. high blood pressure　　（　　　　）
10. appropriate amount　　（　　　　）量

Unit 6 Knowing Your Nutrients
栄養素を知ろう

Vocabulary Check

（　　　）に入る語を下から選びなさい。

1. chemical (　　　　　) 化学組成物
2. (　　　　　) compound 有機化合物
3. element (　　　　　) 炭素
4. (　　　　　) activity 胃腸の活動
5. bodily (　　　　　) 身体機能
6. (　　　　　) compound 無機化合物
7. (　　　　　) element 基本要素
8. (　　　　　) 排泄
9. animal amino (　　　　　) 動物性アミノ酸
10. (　　　　　) acid chain 脂肪酸鎖

> acid, carbon, composition, excretion, fatty, function, fundamental, gastrointestinal, inorganic, organic

🔊 Track10

Nutrients are chemical compositions that your body uses as building blocks in order to function properly. You need nutrients to breathe, to smile, to watch television — to live healthily and well. Nutrients fall into several classes:

☐ **Proteins:** Proteins are an organic energy source, and they provide the raw materials necessary to build body tissues, such as muscles and organs.

Four out of the six types of nutrients — proteins, fats, carbs, and vitamins — are organic compounds, meaning they contain the element carbon and are derived from living things.

☐ **Fats:** Fats are another source of energy for the body. This organic compound helps with many different functions in the body, including vitamin absorption, hormone production, and normal cell functioning.

☐ **Carbohydrates**: Carbs are the primary source of energy for most organisms. This organic compound is essential for normal brain and gastrointestinal activity and functioning.

☐ **Vitamins**: The fourth and final organic nutrient, vitamins are vital to a large number of bodily functions. Needed in small amounts, they are found in almost all whole foods you eat.

☐ **Minerals**: Solid, inorganic compounds found in most of the foods you consume, minerals are crucial to basic body functions. The range of processes that minerals help regulate and maintain is nearly endless.

☐ **Water**: *The* nutrient, the giver and sustainer of life, water is a fundamental element of all foods you eat, and it is the most important nutrient. The majority of the foods you eat are mostly made of water, you are constantly in need of water due to its continuous excretion, and your body is always looking to replace lost water.

You obtain the majority of your nutrients from the foods you eat, but your body can manufacture some as well. For example, your body can create human proteins from the plant or animal amino acids you consume during dinner, and it can create fatty acid chains from an excess of glucose (a building block of carbohydrates) in your diet. Nutrients that you must get from your food because your body cannot manufacture them are called *essential nutrients*.

Notes

nutrient／栄養素　building block／構成単位　in order to ～／～するために　function／機能する　properly／きちんと　breathe／呼吸する　healthily／健康的に　fall into ～／～に分類される　protein／タンパク質　organic energy source／有機エネルギー源　provide／与える　raw material／原料　tissue／組織　A such as B／たとえばBのようなA　muscle／筋肉　organ／器官，臓器　A out of B／BのうちのA　fat／脂肪　carb／（通例，複数形で）炭水化物（carbohydrate）　meaning／つまり～を意味する　contain／含む　be derived from ～／～から生じる　vitamin absorption／ビタミン吸収　hormone production／ホルモン生成　normal cell functioning／正常な細胞機能　primary source of energy／主要エネルギー源　organism／（微）生物，有機体　essential／重要な　be vital to ～／～にとって不可欠である　a large amount of ～／大量の～　whole food／自然食品　mineral／ミネラル　solid／固体　consume／摂取する　be crucial to ～／～にとってきわめて重要である　basic body function／基本的な身体機能　range／範囲　process／過程　regulate／調整する，制限する　maintain／維持する　sustainer／維持させるもの　the majority of ～／～の大部分，～の大多数　be made of ～／～でできている　constantly／絶えず，常に　be in need of ～／～を必要としている　due to ～／～のため，～が原因で　continuous／継続的な　replace／取って替わる　obtain／得る　manufacture／生産する　～ as well／～もまた　during ～／～の間　excess／過剰　glucose／グルコース，ブドウ糖　essential nutrient／必須栄養素

Exercise

A 音声を聴いて，次の英文の（　）内に適語を記入しなさい。また，完成した英文を日本語に直しなさい。　🔊 Track11

1. (　　) (　　) (　　) lose weight, she started to exercise every day.

2. Many English words (　　) (　　) (　　) Latin.

3. Harmony (　　) (　　) (　　) success in team sports.

4. New students are (　　) (　　) (　　) a lot of care and support.

B 和文に合うように，（　）内の語句を並べかえて英文を作りなさい。

1. 良いタンパク源には，肉，卵，豆のような食品が含まれる。
 (as, beans, foods, and, good sources of protein, such, eggs, include, meat).

2. 日本人の4人にひとりは65歳以上だ。
 (65 years old, one, over, Japanese people, of, are, four, out).

3. その患者は大量に出血した。
 (blood, lost, amount, the patient, of, large, a).

Unit 7 Energizing Nutrients: Proteins, Carbs, and Fats
エネルギーの源：タンパク質，炭水化物，脂肪

Vocabulary Check

（　　）に入る語を下から選びなさい。
1. internal (　　　　) 内部体温
2. (　　　　) 分子
3. (　　　　) bond 化学結合
4. (　　　　) 消化
5. peptide (　　　　) ペプチド結合
6. energy (　　　　) エネルギー産生栄養素
7. balanced (　　　　) バランスの取れた食事
8. (　　　　) food 無脂肪食品
9. (　　　　) 消費
10. (　　　　) 栄養補助食品

> bond, chemical, diet, digestion, expenditure, fat-free, molecule, nutrient, supplement, temperature

🔊 Track12

Every single thing you do (walk, laugh, or pick up sticks) or your body does without your direction (breath, regulate internal temperature, and so on) requires energy, and that energy comes from certain food sources: carbohydrates, fats, and proteins. In other words, the energy required for you to read these words came from the bacon and eggs you may have eaten this morning for breakfast; this energy allows you to open this book, turn the pages, read the text, and comprehend the material.

All carbs are just chains of glucose molecules held together by chemical bonds. When those bonds are broken down by digestion, they release energy, called *food energy*. Fats (three fatty acid chains connected into a triglyceride), proteins (chains of amino acids connected by peptide bonds), and carbs all have this property; they are the *energy nutrients*. Here are the things you need to know about these nutrients:

- [ ] Carbs should supply 50 percent to 60 percent of your daily caloric needs, by far the largest supplier. Fats are the next highest supplier of energy for a healthy diet; they should provide approximately 25 percent to 30 percent of your daily energy needs. Proteins are the lowest supplier and should provide around 15 percent to 20 percent of your needed daily calories.

- [ ] A diverse and balanced diet provides a rich source of energy from foods like wheat (carbs), beef (protein), cheese (protein and fat), and so on. Having too much of one source is unhealthy and can pose adverse health problems in the future.

- [ ] When you eat too much energy, your body stores it as fat. Even fat-free foods may be high in calories (think of soft drinks) and can contribute to weight gain if you eat them in excess. Refer to the earlier unit "Keeping Caloric Intake in Check" and the formula for caloric intake and expenditure for information about keeping your body weight stabilized. Bottom line: Try not to overconsume energy nutrients.

You may have heard, or perhaps believe, that vitamins, particularly the B vitamins, are a good source of energy. Don't believe the hype. Many energy supplements claim that they can give you hours and hours of "natural" energy via B vitamins. The problem is that B vitamins *metabolize* energy: they don't *provide* energy. If you don't eat energy nutrients (carbs, fats, and proteins), the B vitamins do little to give you that boost you paid for.

Notes

energizing／エネルギーを与える　nutrient／栄養素　protein／タンパク質　carb／(通例, 複数形で)炭水化物 (carbohydrate)　fat／脂肪　every single ～／あらゆる～　pick up ～／～を拾い上げる　direction／指示, 命令　regulate／調整する　～ and so on／～など　require／必要とする　carbohydrate／炭水化物　in other words／言い換えれば　allow A to ～／Aが～するのを可能にする　comprehend／理解する　material／教材　glucose／グルコース, ブドウ糖　hold together ～／～をまとめる, ～を結合させる　break down ～／～を分解する　release／放出する　food energy／食物エネルギー　fatty acid／脂肪酸　triglyceride／トリグルセリド　amino acid／アミノ酸　property／特性　supply／供給する　by far／(最上級を強めて) 断然　approximately／約, およそ　around／約, およそ　diverse／多様な　wheat／小麦　pose／引き起こす　adverse／有害な　in the future／将来　store／蓄える　think of ～／～を思い起こす　contribute to ～／～の原因となる　weight gain／体重増加　in excess／過度に　refer to ～／～を参照する　keep ～ in check／～を管理する, ～を抑制する　formula／公式　caloric intake／カロリー摂取　stabilize／安定させる　bottom line／肝心な点　overconsume／過剰摂取する　hype／誇大広告　claim／主張する　hours and hours of ～／何時間もの～　the problem is that ～／問題は～である　metabolize／新陳代謝させる　do little to ～／～することにほとんど効果がない　give you that boost you paid for／代金を支払った分だけあなたを元気づける (give ～ a boost は「～を元気づける」)

Exercise

A 音声を聴いて，次の英文の（　　）内に適語を記入しなさい。また，完成した英文を日本語に直しなさい。

🔊 Track13

1. Don't (　　　) (　　　) the foods you dropped.

2. He is (　　　) (　　　) the most popular chef.

3. Please (　　　) (　　　) our website for further information.

4. The (　　　) (　　　) is that we need regular exercise.

B 和文に合うように，（　　）内の語句を並べかえて英文を作りなさい。

1. この製品を使えば短時間で調理できる。
   (cook, short, allows, time, this product, you, in, to, a).

2. 砂糖の過剰摂取は健康によくない。
   (is, sugar, healthy, excess, eating, not, in).

3. 問題は，彼が野菜と果物の摂取不足ということである。
   (consume, problem, he, fruits, is, and, doesn't, vegetables, the, that, enough).

Unit 8 Aiding in Body Function: Vitamins and Minerals
身体機能を助ける：ビタミンとミネラル

Vocabulary Check

（　　）に入る語を下から選びなさい。

1. (　　　　　) 肝臓
2. fatty (　　　　　) 脂肪組織
3. (　　　　　) functioning　免疫システム機能
4. blood (　　　　　) 血管
5. blood (　　　　　) 血中脂質
6. sensory (　　　　　) 感覚神経
7. (　　　　　) contraction　筋収縮
8. (　　　　　) acid　胃酸
9. (　　　　　) 代謝
10. whole (　　　　　) 全粒穀物

> grains, immune-system, lipid, liver, metabolism, muscle, nerve, stomach, tissue, vessel

🔊 Track14

Distinguishing between water-soluble and fat-soluble vitamins

Vitamins come in two classifications:

☐ **Water-soluble (vitamins B and C):** With water-soluble vitamins, your body metabolizes what it needs, and then you urinate the rest out. Because your body doesn't store these vitamins in any large capacity, toxicity is rare. However, because your body easily excretes water-soluble vitamins, you have to make sure you get enough in your diet.

The exception is vitamin B_6, which your body does not excrete as easily. Be careful not to exceed the upper limit of this nutrient.

- **Fat-soluble (vitamins A, D, E, and K):** Fat-soluble vitamins are stored in the liver and fatty tissues and are not as easily excreted by the body as water-soluble vitamins. For these reasons, taking supplements is not necessary unless your doctor directs you to do so. If you're not careful about how much of the fat-soluble vitamins you are ingesting, they can become toxic.

You need fat in your diet to metabolize fat-soluble vitamins. If you take a supplement and eat fat-free foods, you're wasting your money because your body won't be able to use those expensive fat-soluble vitamin supplements.

Vitamins don't cure diseases (other than diseases caused by vitamin deficiencies, of course). For example, drinking orange juice to obtain vitamin C won't cure a cold. The vitamin C may assist in healthy immune-system functioning, but the vitamin alone doesn't cure the disease. On the other hand, drinking orange juice does help cure scurvy, a disease caused by the lack of vitamin C.

Minding your minerals

Minerals — solid, inorganic compounds found in food — are crucial to basic body functions and make up about 5 pounds (2.27 kilograms) of your body weight. The majority of your body's minerals lies in your bones and consists of calcium and phosphorus. Here are the details on these and other key minerals:

- **Calcium:** Found in milk and dairy products and leafy, green vegetables, calcium is crucial for bone development, blood vessel health, and brain activity.

- **Phosphorus:** Found in dairy products, beans, and various fruits and vegetables, phosphorus assists with bone and teeth development, DNA/RNA health, and blood lipid creation.

- **Potassium:** Found in sources such as honeydew melons, citrus fruits, potatoes, and bananas, this mineral is central to healthy cell functioning and blood pressure regulation.

- **Sodium:** By balancing fluids in the body and assisting in proper sensory nerve and muscle contraction functioning, sodium is highly influential on raising blood pressure. Because salt is the major source of sodium, you must be careful not to overconsume high-salt foods.

- ☐ **Sulfur:** Used for treating skin conditions and essential for amino acid manufacturing, this mineral is found in eggs, onions, garlic, and cabbage.

- ☐ **Chloride:** Chloride is crucial for digestion, serving as a fundamental element in the creation of stomach acid. It's found in salt, tomatoes, lettuce, celery, and other vegetables.

- ☐ **Magnesium:** Essential in metabolism and blood pressure regulation, magnesium is found in whole grains and beans.

Notes

distinguish between A and B／AとBを区別する　water-soluble／水溶性の　fat-soluble／脂溶性の　classification／分類　metabolize／新陳代謝させる　urinate／排尿させる　store／蓄える　capacity／容量　toxicity／毒性　excrete／排出する　make sure 〜／必ず〜であるように気をつける　exception／例外　exceed／超える　not as 〜 as ...／…ほど〜でない　supplement／栄養補助食品　unless〜／〜でない限り　direct A to 〜／Aに〜するよう指示する　ingest／摂取する　toxic／毒性の　fat-free／無脂肪の　be able to〜／〜できる　cure／治療する　other than 〜／〜以外の　deficiency／不足，欠乏　obtain／得る　〜 alone／〜のみ　on the other hand／一方で，他方では　scurvy／壊血病　lack／不足　solid／固体の，固形の　inorganic compound／無機化合物　crucial／きわめて重要な　make up 〜／〜を構成する，〜を占める　consist of 〜／〜で構成される　calcium／カルシウム　phosphorus／リン　dairy product／乳製品　leafy／葉からなる　potassium／カリウム　A such as B／たとえばBのようなA　honeydew melon／甘露メロン　citrus fruit／柑橘類　central／中心となる，重要な　blood pressure／血圧　regulation／調節　sodium／ナトリウム　fluid／体液　influential／影響を及ぼす　overconsume／過剰摂取する　sulfur／硫黄　treat／治療する　essential／重要な　amino acid／アミノ酸　manufacturing／生成　chloride／塩化物　digestion／消化　fundamental element／基本要素　magnesium／マグネシウム

Exercise

A 音声を聴いて，次の英文の（　　）内に適語を記入しなさい。また，完成した英文を日本語に直しなさい。

Track15

1. We are looking for a person who (　　　) (　　　) (　　　) communicate well in English.

2. (　　　) (　　　) English, she can speak French and German.

3. I like the color of this jacket. The design, (　　　) (　　　) (　　　) (　　　), is old-fashioned.

4. It (　　　) mainly (　　　) vegetables and rice.

B 和文に合うように，（　　）内の語句を並べかえて英文を作りなさい。

1. 1日を元気に過ごすために，朝食は必ず食べてください。
   (to, the, eat, throughout, sure, stay, day, you, energized, make, breakfast).

2. そのレシピは見かけほど簡単ではない。
   (not, looks, as, is, it, easy, the recipe, as).

3. バランスの取れた食事を摂取しない限り，健康にはなれません。
   (a, can't, eat, unless, diet, be, balanced, you, healthy, you).

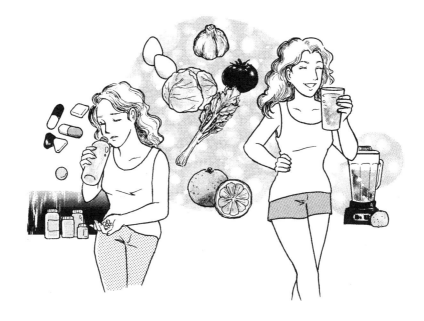

Unit 9 Water: The Most Important Nutrient
水：最も重要な栄養素

Vocabulary Check

（　　　）に入る語を下から選びなさい。

1. (　　　　　　) 関節
2. (　　　　　　) 老廃物
3. (　　　　　　) cord　脊髄
4. (　　　　　　) water　炭酸水
5. (　　　　　　) 尿
6. (　　　　　　) 液体，水分
7. (　　　　　　) 脱水（症）
8. (　　　　　　) 目まい
9. (　　　　　　) 疲労
10. (　　　　　　) failure　腎不全

> carbonated, dehydration, dizziness, exhaustion, fluid, joint, kidney, spinal, urine, waste

---

🔊 Track16

　Thirsty? Grab a cold one. That's right. A nice, tall, cold glass of water. Water is *the* nutrient of all nutrients. You need it to live. Water is so essential that you can't live much more than three days without it. You can live for a month or so without food but not even a week without water.

　Other than slaking thirst, your body needs water to perform these functions:

- ☐ Regulate body temperature
- ☐ Cushion the joints (knee, shoulder, elbow, and so on)
- ☐ Remove bodily waste
- ☐ Protect your spinal cord

How much water you need depends on your activity level, your age, and what you're eating. Ideally, in a given day, you should drink the same amount of water that you lose. Figuring out precisely how much that is is pretty difficult, given that you lose water in many different ways. You even lose water when you exhale! As a general rule, if you drink a glass or two of water with every meal, you'll be fine.

The most obvious way to get the water you need is to drink it. However, you also get water from the foods you eat. That apple you may have eaten for lunch is mostly water. And that bottle of soda you drank last night is mostly carbonated water. You even get water from the turkey sandwich you may be eating right now reading this book.

Having a diet full of fruits and vegetables, drinking water with your meals, and making sure to drink water before, during, and especially after exercising ensures you're staying hydrated! One way to tell that you're staying adequately hydrated is to look at the color of your urine. It should be a pale yellow color. If it's dark yellow, increase your water intake.

Make sure you drink enough fluids throughout the day. Dehydration can lead to many health problems, like dizziness and exhaustion, but if it's persistent, it can lead to kidney failure, coma, and death. Also keep this in mind: When you feel thirsty, you're already dehydrated. So get drinking!

Notes

nutrient／栄養素　thirsty／のどが渇いた　grab／素早く飲む　cold one／冷たい飲み物　so 〜 that ...／とても〜なので…　essential／重要な　〜 or so／〜かそのくらい　other than 〜／〜以外に　slake／(渇きを)いやす　function／機能　regulate／調整する　cushion／和らげる　〜 and so on／〜など　remove／取り除く　depend on 〜／〜による，〜次第である　what you're eating／食べているもの　in a given day／ある特定の日に　the same A that B／Bと同じA　figure out 〜／〜を算定する　precisely／正確に　given that 〜／もし〜と仮定すると　exhale／(息を)吐き出す　as a general rule／一般に，普通は　obvious／明らかな　may have eaten／(may have 過去分詞の形で)食べたかもしれない　right now／ちょうど今　full of 〜／〜でいっぱいの　make sure to 〜／確実に〜する，忘れずに〜する　ensure／確実にする　stay hydrated／(水分補給によって)脱水状態にならないでいる　tell／見分ける　adequately／適切に，十分に　pale yellow／淡黄色　dark yellow／暗黄色　intake／摂取　lead to 〜／〜をもたらす，〜につながる　persistent／持続性の　coma／昏睡　keep 〜 in mind／〜に留意する，〜を覚えておく　dehydrated／脱水状態の　get 〜ing／〜しはじめる

Exercise

A 音声を聴いて，次の英文の（　　）内に適語を記入しなさい。また，完成した英文を日本語に直しなさい。

🔊 Track17

1. Pay attention to (　　　　) (　　　　) (　　　　) (　　　　) (　　　　).

2. I can't (　　　　) (　　　　) the total cost of lunch.

3. I'm working (　　　　) (　　　　).

4. My bag was (　　　　) (　　　　) books.

B 和文に合うように，（　　）内の語句を並べかえて英文を作りなさい。

1. その料理はとても辛かったので，彼女は食べきることができなかった。
   (that, eat, was, she, it, food, couldn't, the, spicy, all, so).

2. 私はおかゆに塩を入れ過ぎたかもしれない。
   (in, have, porridge, too, I, salt, may, the, put, much).

3. 1日の摂取カロリーに留意してください。
   (intake, the, in, keep, calorie, mind, daily).

Unit 10
Binge Drinking: A Behavioral No-No
むちゃ飲み：絶対にやってはならない行為

+Review

🔊 Track18

Binge drinkers have been described as "once-in-a-while alcoholics." They don't drink every day, but when they do indulge, they go so far overboard that they sometimes fail to come back up. In simple terms, binge drinking is downing very large amounts of alcohol in a short time, not for a pleasant lift but to get drunk. As a result, binge drinkers may consume so much beer, wine, or spirits that the amount of alcohol in their blood rises to lethal levels that, in the worst case, may lead (　1　) death by alcohol poisoning.

Efforts to stamp out binge drinking, which often occurs on college campuses, may rely (　2　) guilt or shame to change behavior, but a 2008 study at the Kellogg School of Management at Northwestern University found that binge drinkers are already uncomfortable with their behavior. Attempting to make them more so doesn't work. Instead, the researchers suggested couching anti-binge messages in simple, intelligent language focusing on how to avoid situations that lead to binge drinking rather (　3　) the nasty effects of the overindulgence.

As in other areas of modern life, money matters here, at least to grown-ups. In 2015, scientists at Boston University's School of Public Health published a report in the journal *Addiction*, showing that a simple 1 percent increase in the tax on alcohol beverages lowered the proportion of adult binge drinkers by 1.4 percent. To prove the point, they noted that Tennessee, with the highest taxes on beer, has the lowest proportion of binge drinkers, while states with lower taxes — specifically Delaware, Montana, and Wisconsin — have the highest.

Notes

binge drinking／むちゃ飲み　behavioral／行動に関する　no-no／禁じられたこと　binge drinker／むちゃ飲みする人　"once-in-a-while alcoholic"／「たまに大酒を飲む人」　indulge／大酒を飲む　go overboard／やり過ぎる　so ～ that ...／とても～なので…　fail to ～／～できない　come back up／回復する　term／言い方　down／飲む　amount／量　not A but B／AではなくてB　lift／（精神の）高揚　as a result／その結果として　consume／飲む　spirits／（複数形で）蒸留酒　lethal／致命的な　alcohol poisoning／アルコール中毒　stamp out ～／～を根絶する　guilt／罪悪感　shame／羞恥心　Kellogg School of Management at Northwestern University／（米国イリノイ州エバンストンにある）ノースウェスタン大学ケロッグ経営大学院　uncomfortable／心地よくない　attempt to ～／～することを試みる　work／役に立つ，うまくいく　researcher／研究者　couch／言い表す　anti-binge／反むちゃ飲みの　nasty／厄介な　effect／影響　overindulgence／ふけりすぎ，耽溺　matter／重要である，問題となる　at least／少なくとも　grown-up／成人　Boston University's School Of Public Health／（米国マサチューセッツ州ボストンにある）ボストン大学公衆衛生大学院　*Addiction*／『アディクション』（Society for the Study of Addictionが1884年に創刊した雑誌，addictionは「常用癖，中毒，依存症」）　lower／下げる　proportion／割合　prove／証明する　Tennessee／（米国南東部の）テネシー州　specifically／特に　Delaware／（米国東部の）デラウェア州　Montana／（米国北西部の）モンタナ州　Wisconsin／（米国北中部の）ウィスコンシン州

Exercise

A 英文中の次の語を日本語に直しなさい。

1. blood （　　　　　）
2. behavior （　　　　　）
3. avoid （　　　　　）
4. tax （　　　　　）
5. state （　　　　　）

B 英文中の（　）内に入る語を下から選びなさい。

1. （　　　　　）
2. （　　　　　）
3. （　　　　　）

than, to, on

C 下線部を日本語に直しなさい。

Review (Unit 6〜Unit 9)

A 英文の（ ）内に入る語を下から選んで記入し，英文を日本語に直しなさい。

1. The problems we face fall ( ) three categories. (Unit 6)

2. We talked for hours about our children, our jobs, and so ( ). (Unit 7)

3. Eleven players make ( ) the team. (Unit 8)

4. Make sure ( ) lock the front door. (Unit 9)

> up,　on,　into,　to

B 和文に合うように，（ ）内の語句を並べかえて英文をつくりなさい。

1. 栄養士たちの大多数がその新しい指針に賛成した。(Unit 6)
   (dieticians, the new guidelines, with, of, agreed, the majority).

2. 喫煙とアルコールが彼の早死の原因だった可能性がある。(Unit 7)
   (have, to, early death, contributed, smoking and alcohol, his, could).

3. あの少年は善悪の区別がつかない。(Unit 8)
   (wrong, between, that boy, right, distinguish, cannot, and).

4. 一般に女性は男性よりも長生きだ。(Unit 9)
   (live, men, rule, a, longer, women, general, than, as).

C 次の英語を日本語に直しなさい。

1. raw material　　（　　　　）
2. vitamin absorption　　ビタミン（　　　　）
3. digestion　　（　　　　）
4. wheat　　（　　　　）
5. liver　　（　　　　）
6. immune system　　（　　　　）システム
7. stomach acid　　（　　　　）酸
8. spinal cord　　（　　　　）
9. dehydration　　（　　　　）
10. kidney　　（　　　　）

Unit 11 Digestion: One Step at a Time
消化：一歩ずつ着実に

Vocabulary Check

（　　）に入る語を下から選びなさい。

1. (　　　　) 器官，臓器
2. (　　　　) 胃
3. small (　　　　) 小腸
4. (　　　　) 鼻孔
5. salivary (　　　　) 唾液腺
6. (　　　　) 分泌する
7. (　　　　) 食道
8. (　　　　) 筋肉
9. (　　　　) 収縮
10. (　　　　) 酵素
11. hydrochloric (　　　　) 塩酸
12. (　　　　) 粘液
13. (　　　　) 成分
14. (　　　　) 結腸

> acid, colon, contraction, enzyme, esophagus, gland, ingredient, intestine, mucus, muscle, nostril, organ, secrete, stomach

Track19

Each organ in the digestive system plays a specific role in the digestive drama. But the first act occurs in three places rarely listed as part of the digestive tract: your brain, your eyes, and your nose. The next acts take place in your mouth, your stomach, and your small and large intestines.

Your brain, eyes, and nose

When you see appetizing food, you experience a conditioned response. In other words, your thoughts — "Wow! That looks good!" — stimulate your brain to tell your digestive organs to get ready for action.

What happens in your nose is purely physical. The tantalizing aroma of good food is transmitted by molecules that fly from the surface of the food to settle on the membrane lining of your nostrils; these molecules stimulate the receptor cells on the olfactory nerve fibers that stretch from your nose back to your brain. When the receptor cells communicate with your brain, your brain sends encouraging messages to your mouth and digestive tract as the sight and scent of food make your mouth water and your stomach contract in anticipatory hunger pangs.

Your mouth

Lift your fork to your mouth, and your teeth and salivary glands swing into action. Your teeth chew, grinding and breaking food into small, manageable pieces.

At the same time, salivary glands under your tongue and in the back of your mouth secrete the watery liquid called *saliva*, which performs two important functions.

Your stomach

If you were to lay your digestive tract out on a table, most of it would look like a simple, rather narrow, tube. The exception is your stomach, a pouchlike structure just below your esophagus.

Like most of the digestive tube, your stomach is circled with strong muscles whose rhythmic peristaltic contractions turn your stomach into a sort of food processor that mechanically breaks pieces of food into ever smaller particles. While this is going on, glands in the stomach wall are secreting *stomach juices* — a potent blend of enzymes, hydrochloric acid, and mucus.

Your small intestine

Open your hand and put it flat against your belly button, with your thumb pointing up to your waist and your little finger pointing down.

Your hand is now covering most of the relatively small space into which your 20-foot-long small intestine is neatly coiled. When the partially digested chyme spills from your stomach into this part of the digestive tube, a whole new set of gastric juices are released.

While these chemicals work, contractions of the small intestine continue to move the food mass down through the tube so your body can absorb sugars, amino acids, fatty acids, vitamins, and minerals into cells in the intestinal wall.

Your large intestine

When every useful, digestible ingredient other than water has been wrung out of your food, the rest — indigestible waste such as fiber — moves into the top of your large intestine, the area known as your *colon*. The colon's primary job is to absorb water from this mixture and then to squeeze the remaining matter into the compact bundle known as feces.

Notes

digestion／消化　digestive system／消化(器)系　play a role in ～／～で役割を果たす　act／幕　rarely／めったに～しない　digestive tract／消化管　take place／起こる，行われる　large intestine／大腸　appetizing／食欲をそそるような　conditioned response／条件反応　in other words／言い換えれば　stimulate／刺激する　digestive organ／消化器官　get ready for ～／～の準備をする　tantalizing／興味をそそる　transmit／伝達する　molecule／分子　settle／おりる　membrane lining／粘膜の層　receptor cell／受容器細胞　olfactory nerve fiber／嗅神経線維　encouraging／奨励する　scent／匂い　water／よだれが出る　contract／収縮する　anticipatory／予期しての　hunger pang／空腹痛　Lift your fork to your mouth, and …／（命令文＋and …の形で）～しなさい，そうすれば…　swing into action／すばやく行動を起こす　chew／噛む　grind／細かく砕く　manageable／処理しやすい　at the same time／同時に　saliva／唾液　If you were to ～／（条件を表すif節の中でbe to ～）もし～するつもりならば　lay ～ out／～を広げる　exception／例外　pouchlike／袋のような形をした　structure／構造　digestive tube／消化管　be circled with ～／～で囲まれる　peristaltic／蠕動性の　particle／小さな粒　go on／続く　gland／腺　stomach wall／胃壁　stomach juice／胃液　potent／強い，濃い　blend／混合物　flat／平らに　belly button／へそ　relatively／比較的　20-foot-long／長さ20フィート（約6.1メートル）の　neatly／きちんと　partially／部分的に　digest／消化する　chyme／糜粥　spill／こぼれる，溢れる　gastric juice／胃液　release／放出する　chemical／化学物質　mass／塊　so your body can absorb／（so (that) A can ～の形で）Aが～するために　absorb／吸収する　sugar／糖　amino acid／アミノ酸　fatty acid／脂肪酸　intestinal wall／腸壁　digestible／消化できる，消化しやすい　other than ～／～以外の　wring A out of B／AをBから搾り取る　the rest／残り　indigestible／消化できない，消化しにくい　A such as B／たとえばBのようなA　fiber／食物繊維　mixture／混合物　squeeze／絞る　remaining／残りの　matter／物質　compact／緻密な　bundle／束　feces／糞便

===== Exercise =====

A 音声を聴いて，次の英文の（　）内に適語を記入しなさい。また，完成した英文を日本語に直しなさい。
🔊 Track20

1. The meeting will (　　　) (　　　) on Wednesday.

2. The twins are (　　　) (　　　) (　　　) bed.

3. Doctors have already (　　　) (　　　) (　　　).

4. I can't concentrate on two things (　　　) (　　　) (　　　) (　　　).

B 和文に合うように，（　）内の語句を並べかえて英文を作りなさい。

1. 親は子どもの食育で重要な役割を果たす。
   (in, important, children's food and nutrition education, play, parents, role, an, their).

2. 角を左へ曲がりなさい，そうすれば食品加工プラントがあります。
   (find, at, and, a food processing plant, the corner, you'll, left, turn).

3. 弁当を作るために早起きしなければならない。
   (can, early, I, a box lunch, get up, so, have to, prepare, I).

Unit 12 Eating Disorders
摂食障害

Vocabulary Check

（　　　）に入る語を下から選びなさい。
1. (　　　) 食欲
2. psychological (　　　) 心理的苦痛
3. (　　　) 関節炎
4. (　　　) 糖尿病
5. (　　　) 飢餓
6. (　　　) cycle 月経周期
7. (　　　) 緩下薬，通じ薬
8. (　　　) 催吐薬
9. (　　　) 胃
10. (　　　) カリウム
11. heart (　　　) 心不全
12. (　　　) 診断
13. (　　　) 栄養不良

> appetite, arthritis, diabetes, diagnosis, distress, emetic, failure, laxative, malnutrition, menstrual, potassium, starvation, stomach

Track21

For some people, food is not simply a meal. It is the object of love or loathing, a way to relieve anxiety or an anxiety provoker. As a result, human beings may experience various eating disorders — *obesity, anorexia nervosa, bulimia, and binge eating* — which I describe in the following sections.

Obesity

Although everyone knows that there's a worldwide increase in obesity, not everyone who is larger or heavier than the current ideal body has an eating disorder. Human bodies come in many different sizes, and some healthy people are just naturally larger or heavier than others. But an eating disorder may be present when

- [ ] A person continually confuses the desire for food (appetite) with the need for food (hunger)

- [ ] A person who has access to a normal diet experiences psychological distress when denied food

- [ ] A person uses food to relieve anxiety provoked by what he or she considers a scary situation — a new job, a party, ordinary criticism, or a deadline

Traditionally, doctors find it difficult to treat obesity, but in recent years, some studies have suggested that some people overeat in response to irregularities in the production of chemicals that regulate satiety (the feeling of fullness). This research may open the path to new kinds of drugs that can control extreme appetite, thus reducing the incidence of obesity-related disorders, such as arthritis, diabetes, high blood pressure, and heart disease.

Anorexia nervosa

Anorexia is voluntary starvation. As you may expect, anorexia is virtually unknown in places where food is hard to come by. Instead, this condition is often considered an affliction of affluence, most likely to strike the young and well-to-do, men as well as women, although more commonly women.

The signs of anorexia are weight less than 85 percent of the normal weight, a fear of gaining weight, an obsession with one's appearance, and the belief that one is fat regardless of the true weight. For young women, anorexia can lead to the absence of menstrual cycles.

Up to 40 percent of people with anorexia develop *bulimia nervosa*; up to 30 percent develop *binge eating disorder*, the next two problems in this unit. Left untreated, anorexia nervosa may be fatal.

Bulimia nervosa

Unlike people with anorexia, individuals with bulimia don't refuse to eat, but they don't want to hold on to the food they've consumed. They may use laxatives to increase defecation, or they may simply retire to the bathroom after eating to take *emetics* (drugs that induce vomiting) or stick their fingers into their throats to make themselves throw up. Like anorexics, bulimics may develop *binge eating disorder*.

Either way, danger looms. Repeated regurgitation can severely irritate or even tear through the lining of the esophagus (throat). Acidic stomach contents also damage teeth, which is why dentists are often the first medical personnel to identify a bulimic. Finally, the continued use of emetics may result in a life-threatening loss of potassium that triggers irregular heartbeat or heart failure.

Binge eating disorder

The criterion for a diagnosis of binge eating disorder is consuming enormous amounts of food — a whole chicken, several pints of ice cream, an entire loaf of bread — in one sitting twice a week for up to six months. Some binge eaters become overweight; others stay slim by regurgitating. Either way, binge eating, like other eating disorders, is hazardous behavior.

Binge eaters who regurgitate experience adverse effects similar to those associated with bulimia. Binge eaters who don't regurgitate risk not only obesity but also, paradoxically, malnutrition. Why? Because the foods they choose may be high in calories but low in vital nutrients. (Think hot fudge sundae again, and again, and again.) More dramatically, the enormous quantities of food they consume may dilate or even rupture the stomach or esophagus, a potentially fatal medical emergency.

Unit 13 Food Allergies
食物アレルギー

Vocabulary Check

（　　　）に入る語を下から選びなさい。

1. （　　　　　）細菌
2. （　　　　　）抗体
3. （　　　　　）蕁麻疹性丘疹
4. （　　　　　）痒み
5. （　　　　　）腫れあがり
6. （　　　　　）発疹
7. （　　　　　）偏頭痛
8. （　　　　　）吐き気
9. （　　　　　）嘔吐
10. （　　　　　）下痢
11. （　　　　　）組織
12. white blood （　　　　　）白血球
13. gastrointestinal （　　　　　）胃腸管
14. （　　　　　）症状
15. （　　　　　）鎮痛薬

> analgesic, antibody, bacteria, cell, diarrhea, hives, itching, migraine, nausea, rash, swelling, symptom, tissue, tract, vomiting

🔊 Track23

Your immune system is designed to protect your body from harmful invaders, such as bacteria. Sometimes, however, the system responds to substances normally considered harmless. The substance that provokes the attack is called an *allergen*; the substances that attack the allergen are called *antibodies*.

A food allergy can provoke such a response as your body releases antibodies to attack specific proteins in food. When this happens, some of the physical reactions include

- [ ] Hives
- [ ] Itching
- [ ] Swelling of the face, tongue, lips, eyelids, hands, and feet
- [ ] Rashes
- [ ] Headaches, migraines
- [ ] Nausea and/or vomiting
- [ ] Diarrhea, sometimes bloody
- [ ] Sneezing, coughing
- [ ] Asthma
- [ ] Breathing difficulties caused by *tightening* (swelling) of tissues in the throat
- [ ] Loss of consciousness (from anaphylactic shock)

If you're sensitive to a specific food, you may not have to eat the food to have the reaction. For example, people sensitive to peanuts may break out in hives just from touching a peanut or peanut butter and may suffer a potentially fatal reaction after tasting chocolate that has touched factory machinery that previously touched peanuts. People sensitive to seafood — fin fish and shellfish — have been known to develop breathing problems after simply inhaling the vapors or steam produced by cooking the fish.

Understanding how an allergic reaction occurs

When you eat food containing a protein to which you're sensitive, the protein reaches antibodies on the surface of white blood cells called *basophils* and immune system cells called *mast cells* either in your gastrointestinal tract or by circulating through the bloodstream.

The basophils and mast cells produce, store, and release *histamine*, a natural body chemical that causes the symptoms — itching, swelling, hives — associated with allergic reactions (some allergy pills designed to counter this are called *antihistamines*). When the antibodies on the surface of the basophils and mast cells come in contact with food allergens, the cells release histamine, and the result is an *allergic reaction.*

Most allergic reactions to food are unpleasant but essentially mild. However, as many as 150 or more people die every year in the United States from a severe reaction to a food allergen.

Coping with Food Allergies

To keep yourself or your allergic friends and family safe in a world practically teeming with allergens, know what's in your food, check out unusual allergenic couplings, work with others to make rules that work, and practice simple protection.

Reading the food ingredient label

According to the Food Allergy and Anaphylaxis Network, more than 90 percent of all allergic reactions to foods are caused by just eight foods; eggs, fish, milk, peanuts, shellfish, soy, tree nuts, and wheat.

If you're sensitive to one of these foods, the best way to avoid an allergic reaction is to avoid the food. And you can do that by reading the label to ferret out hidden ingredients — peanuts in the chili or caviar (fish eggs) in the dip.

Avoiding unusual interactions

Sometimes a food label doesn't list an allergen because the allergen is simply (surprise!) a natural component of the food.

Salicylates are a perfect example. These natural chemicals occur in many plants, including some plants that end up on the dinner table. The salicylates protect the plants by destroying mold and other microorganisms. For human beings, salicylates act as analgesics (pain killers), the most famous of which is *acetylsalicylic acid*, better known as *aspirin*. People who are sensitive to salicylates may experience an allergic reaction (wheezing and difficulty breathing, headache, hives, rash or itchy skin, and swollen hands, feet, or face) when exposed even to very small amounts, including the salicylates in otherwise highly nutritious plant foods such as fruits and vegetables.

Notes

allergy／アレルギー　immune system／免疫システム　be designed to ～／～するように作られている　harmful／有害な　invader／侵入物　A such as B／たとえばBのようなA　substance／物質　harmless／無害な　provoke／引き起こす　allergen／アレルゲン　such A as B／たとえばBのようなA　release／放出する　specific／特定の　protein／タンパク質　eyelid／瞼　A and/or B／AおよびB、またはいずれか一方　bloody／出血している　sneezing／くしゃみをすること　coughing／咳をすること　asthma／喘息　tightening／ピンと張ること　loss of consciousness／意識消失　anaphylactic shock／アナフィラキシーショック　sensitive／過敏な　break out in ～／（発疹など）～でいっぱいになる，覆われる　suffer／経験する，被る　fatal／致命的な　taste／（ひと口）食べる　machinery／機械類　previously／以前に　fin fish／（shellfishに対してひれのある）魚　shellfish／貝，甲殻類　inhale／吸入する　vapor／蒸気　steam／湯気　allergic reaction／アレルギー反応　surface／表面　basophil／好塩基球　mast cell／マスト細胞　either A or B／AまたはB　circulate／循環する　bloodstream／血流　store／貯蔵する　histamine／ヒスタミン　chemical／化学物質　associated with ～／～と関連した　pill／丸剤，錠剤　counter／対抗する　antihistamine／抗ヒスタミン薬　come in contact with ～／～と接触する　as many as ～／～もの数の　cope with ～／～に対処する　teem with ～／～でいっぱいの　check out ～／～を点検する，調査する　allergenic／アレルゲン性の，アレルギーを誘発する　coupling／結合　ingredient／成分　according to ～／～によれば　Food Allergy and Anaphylaxis Network／食品アレルギー・アナフィラキシー・ネットワーク（1991年に設立され，2012年にはFood Allergy Initiative（1998設立）との統合によりFood Allergy Research & Educationとなった）　soy／大豆　tree nut／木の実　ferret out ～／～を捜し出す　hidden／隠れた　chili／チリコンカルネ（メキシコ料理）　caviar／キャビア　dip／ディップ（クラッカーや野菜などにつけて食べるクリーム状のソース）　salicylate／サリチル酸塩　end up ～／最終的に～になる　mold／カビ　microorganism／微生物　pain killer／鎮痛薬　acetylsalicylic acid／アセチルサリチル酸　aspirin／アスピリン　wheezing／ゼイゼイ息をすること　itchy／痒い　swollen／腫れあがった　otherwise／他の点では　nutritious／栄養分のある

Exercise

A 音声を聴いて，次の英文の（　）内に適語を記入しなさい。また，完成した英文を日本語に直しなさい。
　　Track24

1. He (　　　) (　　　) (　　　) a cold sweat.

2. You can have (　　　) (　　　) (　　　) (　　　).

3. This substance should not (　　　) (　　　) (　　　) (　　　) food.

4. You have to (　　　) (　　　) the nursing home.

B 和文に合うように，（　）内の語句を並べかえて英文を作りなさい。

1. これらの方策は，家庭での食品廃棄物を減らすために作られている。
   (at, designed, food waste, to, home, these measures, reduce, are).

2. 食堂には200人もの学生がいた。
   (200 students, as, were, the cafeteria, many, in, there, as).

3. もし彼女が盗みを続けるなら，最後は刑務所に行くことになるだろう。
   (prison, steal, continues, she'll, if, up, in, she, end, to).

Unit 14 Controlling Food Contamination
食物汚染を食い止めよう

Vocabulary Check

（　　　）に入る語を下から選びなさい。

1. (　　　　　　　) 汚染物質，汚染菌
2. (　　　　　　　) 飲食
3. (　　　　　　　) 微生物，細菌
4. (　　　　　　　) 糞便
5. (　　　　　　　) さらす
6. (　　　　　　　) 殺菌した
7. (　　　　　　　) 環境
8. (　　　　　　　) 交差汚染，二次汚染
9. (　　　　　　　) 台所用品
10. (　　　　　　　) 有害な，危険な

> consumption, contaminant, cross-contamination, environment, expose, feces, hazardous, microbe, sterile, utensil

🔊 Track25

Discovering the prevalence of contamination

　Does your food always have some contaminant in it? Short answer: absolutely. Never, ever, will your food be 100 percent free of natural food contaminants. From the farm to the tableside, your food travels hundreds, perhaps thousands of miles — probably in the back of an 18-wheel rig in a crate for about three or four days — and is touched by many hands, all of which increase the chance that your food product will contain food contamination. Even if you grow your food in your own backyard and personally wash and prepare it yourself for consumption, you still can't completely avoid contaminants.

Recognizing the risks contaminants pose to your health

Will you get sick from food contamination? Short answer: Mostly not. After all, you eat contaminants every day. Slightly lengthier answer: Whether food contaminants make you sick depends on how much of the contaminant you ingest; whether that contaminant is a microbe (virus, bacterium, parasite, and so on); and whether that microbe has toxic qualities.

Taking steps to prevent contamination

Can you prevent contamination? Short answer: No. It's just too easy for contaminants to come into contact with your food. From harvest to table, a nearly infinite number of ways exist for hair, dirt, feces, or whatever to get on or in your food. Whether your food grows in a patch outside your backdoor or in a field in the middle of Iowa or Saskatchewan; travels from a local farmers' market or in the back of a semi-tractor trailer going cross-country; is prepared by Grandma, a fry cook, or a renowned chef at a famous bistro; is delivered to your table by wait staff or your kids; or is exposed at any other point in this process, accidental contaminants can get into your food at any time.

So unless you can grow, transport, prepare, and deliver your food in an absolutely sterile environment, you can bet that you'll eat some contaminants each and every day of your life. Weird, right? So relax. You've been eating these things since you were an infant and will continue to for the rest of your life.

Avoiding cross-contamination

Cross-contamination occurs when food is exposed to microbes in the environment. It occurs when microbes and dirt from people, raw meat, and raw fruits and vegetables come in contact — via hands, utensils, poor storage practices, and so on — with ready-to-eat foods.

You can do the following to prevent cross-contamination:

- ☐ Minimize hand contact with food and wash your hands after touching any raw food.
- ☐ Separate raw and cooked foods.
- ☐ Use separate utensils to handle raw and cooked foods.

The basic idea is to keep raw meat, raw seafood and fish, raw eggs, and untreated water away from cooked vegetables, cooked meat, cooked fish, and ready-to-eat foods like sandwiches, salads, cookies, and so on.

Handling potentially hazardous foods with care

You also need to be mindful of potentially hazardous foods. These foods grow microbes more easily than other foods.

Maintaining safe temperatures for cooked and stored food

Microbial contaminants — particularly bacteria — like things nice and warm. Environments that are either too hot or too cold impede bacterial growth. You can use this knowledge to keep your food safe.

Notes

prevalence／蔓延，流行　absolutely／（質問に対して）全くその通り　never, ever／絶対に〜ない　be free of 〜／〜がない　hundreds of 〜／何百もの〜　thousands of 〜／何千もの〜　18-wheel rig／トレーラートラック　crate／輸送用木箱　contamination／汚染　even if 〜／たとえ〜だとしても　prepare／調理する　not completely 〜／完全に〜というわけではない　pose／引き起こす，もたらす　after all 〜／だって〜だから　lengthy／長く続く，長すぎる　whether 〜／〜かどうか　depend on 〜／〜による，〜次第である　ingest／摂取する　virus／ウイルス　bacterium／細菌（bacteriaの単数形）　parasite／寄生虫　〜 and so on／〜など　toxic／中毒性の，有毒の　take steps／対策を講じる　too 〜 for A to ...／Aが…するのは〜すぎる　come into contact with 〜／〜と接触する　an infinite number of 〜／無数の〜　whether A or B／AであろうとBであろうと　patch／（耕作した）一区画　in the middle of 〜／〜の真ん中の　Iowa／（米国中西部の）アイオワ州　Saskatchewan／（カナダ南西部の）サスカチュワン州　farmers' market／農産物直売所　semi-tractor trailer／セミトレーラー（積載荷物の一部を連結したトラクターにもたせかける方式のトレーラー）　cross-country／全国を横断して　Grandma／おばあちゃん　fry cook／フライ料理専門のコック　renowned／著名な　bistro／小さなレストラン　wait staff／給仕スタッフ　accidental／思いがけない　at any time／いつでも　you can bet that 〜／〜であるのは間違いない　weird／気味の悪い　right?／そうですよね？　infant／幼児　for the rest of one's life／これからずっと　raw／生の，未調理の　come in contact with 〜／〜と接触する　via 〜／〜によって　storage practice／貯蔵習慣　ready-to-eat／すぐに食べられる，インスタントの　minimize／最小限にする　away from 〜／〜から離れて　be mindful of 〜／〜に気をつける　microbial／微生物の，細菌の　bacteria／細菌，バクテリア　impede／妨げる

Exercise

A 音声を聴いて，次の英文の（　）内に適語を記入しなさい。また，完成した英文を日本語に直しなさい。　　　　　　　　　　　　　　　Track26

1. The patient was finally (　　　) (　　　) pain.

2. There were (　　　) (　　　) people at the game.

3. I don't care (　　　) (　　　) (　　　) (　　　) (　　　).

4. The phone rang (　　　) (　　　) (　　　) (　　　) the night.

B 和文に合うように，（　）内の語句を並べかえて英文を作りなさい。

1. たとえ走っても，始発のバスには間に合わないだろう。
   (you, the first bus, run, if, catch, you, even, won't).

2. 彼女はこれからずっと車椅子での生活だろう。(Unit 12)
   (a wheelchair, her life, for, in, she'll, the rest, be, of).

3. 食生活に気をつけてください。
   (your, mindful, habits, of, eating, be).

Unit 15 +Review

The Father of All Vitamins: Casimir Funk

ビタミンの父：カシミール・フンク

🔊 Track27

Vitamins are so much a part of modern life that you may have a hard time believing they were first conclusively identified and defined less (1) a century ago. Of course, people have long known that certain foods contain *something* special. For example, nearly 4,000 years ago, the Egyptian King Amenophis IV consumed liver to help him see clearly when the light was poor; 2,000 years later, the Greek physician Hippocrates prescribed raw liver soaked in honey for *nyctalopia* ("night blindness").

(2) the end of the 18th century (1795), British Navy ships carried a mandatory supply of limes or lime juice to prevent scurvy among the men on long journeys, thus earning the Brits once and forever the nickname "limeys." The Japanese, whose sailors had similar problems with beriberi (from *biribiri*, the word for *weak* in Sinhala, a language spoken in Sri Lanka), protected their men by adding whole grain barley to the normal ship's rations.

Everyone knew these remedies worked, but no one knew why until the turn of the 20th century when Casimir Funk, a Polish biochemist working first in England and then in the United States, identified "somethings" in food that he called *vitamins* (*vita* = life; *amines* = nitrogen compounds).

The following year, Funk and a fellow biochemist, Briton Frederick Hopkins, suggested that some medical conditions, such (3) scurvy and beriberi, were simply deficiency diseases caused by the absence of a specific nutrient in the body. <u>Adding a food with the missing nutrient to one's diet would prevent or cure the deficiency disease.</u> What else is there to say except *Eureka!*

Notes

Casimir Funk／カシミール・フンク (1884-1967)（ビタミンを発見して命名したことで知られるポーランド生まれの生化学者）　so ~ that ...／とても~なので…　have a hard time ~ing／なかなか~できない　conclusively／最終的に　identify／突きとめる　define／明確にする　century／一世紀，100年　certain／（明示を避けて）ある　the Egyptian King Amenophis IV／古代エジプト第18王朝の王アメンホテプ4世　consume／食べる　the Greek physician Hippocrates／ギリシャの医師ヒポクラテス　raw／生の　soak／浸す　*nyctalopia*／夜盲（症），鳥目（＝night blindness）　British Navy／英国海軍　mandatory／必須の　lime／ライム　scurvy／壊血病　earn／もたらす　Brit／英国人　once and forever／きっぱりと（＝once and for all）　"limeys"／（軽蔑的に）英国人　beriberi／脚気　Sinhala／シンハラ語　Sri Lanka／スリランカ　whole grain／全粒穀物　barley／大麦　ration／（複数形で）糧食　remedy／療法　work／効く，役に立つ　until the turn of the 20th century／20世紀の初頭まで　Polish／ポーランド人の　biochemist／生化学者　nitrogen compound／窒素化合物　Briton／英国人　Frederick Hopkins／英国人生化学者フレデリック・ホプキンズ (1861-1947)　deficiency disease／欠乏(性)疾患　missing／欠けている　cure／治療する　What else is there to say except ~／~以外に言うことが他にあるか　*Eureka!*／わかった！，しめた！

Exercise

A 英文中の次の語を日本語に直しなさい。
1. contain　(　　　　　　　)
2. liver　(　　　　　　　)
3. prescribe　(　　　　　　　)
4. prevent　(　　　　　　　)
5. nutrient　(　　　　　　　)

B 英文中の（　）内に入る語を下から選びなさい。
1. (　　　　　　)
2. (　　　　　　)
3. (　　　　　　)

> as,　than,　by

C 下線部を日本語に直しなさい。

Review (Unit 11～Unit 14)

A 英文の（　）内に入る語を下から選んで記入し，英文を日本語に直しなさい。

1. She laid her clothes (　　　　) on the bed. (Unit 11)

2. Do you have access (　　　　) a computer? (Unit 12)

3. These illnesses are associated (　　　　) smoking. (Unit 13)

4. Natural disasters can happen (　　　　) any time. (Unit 14)

> at, to, out, with

B 和文に合うように，（　）内の語句を並べかえて英文をつくりなさい。

1. もし管理栄養士になるつもりなら，熱心に勉強しなければならない。(Unit 11)
   (become, have to, hard, to, you, study, you'll, are, if, a registered dietitian).

2. サッカーが好きな生徒もいれば，バレーボールが好きな生徒もいる。(Unit 12)
   (others, students, and, like, volleyball, soccer, like, some).

3. 天気予報によれば，明日は雪になる。(Unit 13)
   (to, going, tomorrow, the weather report, snow, to, it's, according).

4. そのダイニングテーブルは重すぎてひとりでは運べなかった。(Unit 14)
   (too, one person, heavy, to, the dining table, carry, was, for).

C 次の英語を日本語に直しなさい。
1. small intestine　　小（　　　　）
2. saliva　　（　　　　）
3. enzyme　　（　　　　）
4. diabetes　　（　　　　）
5. diagnosis　　（　　　　）
6. malnutrition　　栄養（　　　　）
7. diarrhea　　（　　　　）
8. asthma　　（　　　　）
9. cross-contamination　　交差（　　　　）
10. sterile　　（　　　　）した

編著者紹介

田中　芳文（たなか　よしふみ）
　1985 年　岡山大学大学院教育学研究科（英語教育専攻）修了
　現　在　島根県立大学人間文化学部教授

著者紹介

中里　菜穂子（なかざと　なおこ）
　2006 年　獨協大学大学院外国語学研究科（英語教育専攻）修了
　現　在　聖徳大学語学教育センター非常勤講師

松浦　加寿子（まつうら　かずこ）
　2000 年　岡山大学大学院教育学研究科（英語教育専攻）修了
　2003 年　広島大学大学院文学研究科（英語学英文学専攻）博士課程
　　　　　後期単位取得満期退学
　現　在　倉敷市立短期大学保育学科准教授

NDC 590　　61p　　26cm

やさしい栄養英語（えいようえいご）

　2019 年 2 月 15 日　第 1 刷発行
　2025 年 2 月 13 日　第 3 刷発行

編著者　田中芳文（たなかよしふみ）
著　者　中里菜穂子・松浦加寿子（なかざとなおこ・まつうらかずこ）
発行者　篠木和久
発行所　株式会社　講談社
　　　　〒112-8001　東京都文京区音羽 2-12-21
　　　　　　販　売　(03) 5395-5817
　　　　　　業　務　(03) 5395-3615
編　集　株式会社　講談社サイエンティフィク
　　　　代表　堀越俊一
　　　　〒162-0825　東京都新宿区神楽坂 2-14　ノービィビル
　　　　　　編　集　(03) 3235-3701
印刷所　株式会社ＫＰＳプロダクツ
製本所　株式会社国宝社

落丁本・乱丁本は，購入書店名を明記のうえ，講談社業務宛にお送りください．送料小社負担にてお取替えいたします．なお，この本の内容についてのお問い合わせは，講談社サイエンティフィク宛にお願いいたします．定価はカバーに表示してあります．

© Y. Tanaka, N. Nakazato and K. Matsuura, 2019

本書のコピー，スキャン，デジタル化等の無断複製は著作権法上での例外を除き禁じられています．本書を代行業者等の第三者に依頼してスキャンやデジタル化することはたとえ個人や家庭内の利用でも著作権法違反です．

Printed in Japan
ISBN978-4-06-513414-6

やさしい英語ニュースで学ぶ
現代社会と健康
田中 芳文・編著
B5・110頁・定価2,640円（税込）

健康・医療・生活のニュースでトレーニングする英語教科書。一般向け記事なので、現代社会とのつながりを意識しながらスラスラ読める。

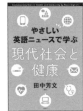

ISBN 978-4-06-155633-1

英文ニュースで学ぶ
健康とライフスタイル
田中 芳文・編著
B5・112頁・定価2,860円（税込）

医療や健康の話題を扱ったニュース記事で英語リーディング能力をレベルアップ！ 一般人向けの記事だから、出てくる用語は一般常識レベルで、文章も読みやすい。看護系や健康栄養系の学生のための新しい英語トレーニング！

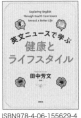

ISBN978-4-06-155629-4

ニュースで読む医療英語
CD付き
川越 栄子・編著
森 茂／田中 芳文／名木田 恵理子／大下 晴美・著
B5・112頁・定価3,080円（税込）

医療・看護のためのやさしい英語テキスト。一般向けのわかりやすい医療ニュースを題材に、入門レベルの読者でもすらすら読める。ネイティブ読み上げCD付きでリスニングもバッチリ！

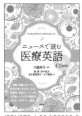

ISBN978-4-06-156310-0

やさしい栄養英語
田中 芳文・編著
中里 菜穂子／松浦 加寿子・著
B5・64頁・定価1,980円（税込）

英語の栄養学読み物を題材にした教科書。一般向けの読み物だから、簡単な英文でスラスラ読める。栄養学の基礎も身についてー石二鳥！
　用語説明も充実しているので、辞書をひく必要なし。英文の長さや問題の量、本全体のページ数に至るまで、スッキリ学べる手ごろな分量。

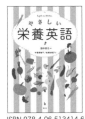

ISBN 978-4-06-513414-6

はじめての栄養英語
えっ、Dietって、やせるって意味じゃないの？
栄養士の私はDietitianなんだ！
美味しく学べる英語のスキル
清水 雅子・著
B5・112頁・定価1,980円（税込）

やさしい英文で初学者でも栄養英語に親しめるよう工夫されたテキスト。栄養素、代謝、解剖生理、消化吸収、食品添加物、食物アレルギーなどを、やさしく短い英文でとりあげた。

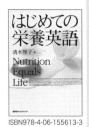

ISBN978-4-06-155613-3

はじめての臨床栄養英語
清水 雅子／J. パトリック・バロン・著
B5・128頁・定価2,530円（税込）

栄養管理を必要とする疾患を中心に、平易な英文で、組織・器官の名称、病気の概要、診断基準、食事療法、薬物療法を学ぶ、これまでにない教科書。病院臨地実習やゼミで必須となる基本英語を集約。大学院受験にも役立つ1冊。

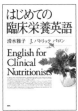

ISBN978-4-06-155621-8

Let's Study English!
Health and Nutrition
英語で読む健康と栄養
横尾 信男・編著
A5・96頁・定価1,650円（税込）

栄養系学生のための教職課程英語テキスト。健康な食生活に必要な知識（栄養素やその摂取法、病気にならない食生活・エクササイズ、酒やタバコの害、食中毒、ストレス解消など）を幅広く学べるように編集。

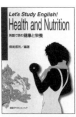

ISBN978-4-06-153951-8

耳から学ぶ
楽しいナース英語
CD付き
中西 睦子・監修　野口 ジュディー／川越 栄子／仁平 雅子・著
B5・112頁・定価3,740円（税込）

CDを聞きながら学ぶ看護英語の決定版。国際化時代の医療現場では英語は不可欠の時代、聞きとれること話せることは必要要素。「どうかしましたか」「どのように痛みますか」こんな会話が話せるようになる1冊。

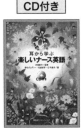

ISBN978-4-06-153672-2

医療従事者のための
医学英語入門
清水 雅子・著
A5・216頁・定価2,750円（税込）

人体組織、器官を中心に基礎医学をコンパクトに収載した1991年刊の好評テキスト『医療技術者のための医学英語入門』が新版となって登場。図版も追加され、さらに使いやすくなった。

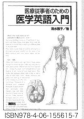

ISBN978-4-06-155615-7

英語で学ぶプライマリーケア
西牟田 祐美子・編著
B5・112頁・定価2,200円（税込）

読んで楽しい看護学生向けテキスト。カラー4コマ漫画を手始めに、看護現場の様子を英語で学ぶことができる。リーディング、文法、演習問題も掲載。リスニング教材をホームページからダウンロード可能。

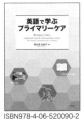

ISBN978-4-06-520090-2

講談社サイエンティフィク https://www.kspub.co.jp/

※表示価格は消費税(10%)が加算されています。

2025年1月現在